Pregnancy Diet Cookbook for Beginners

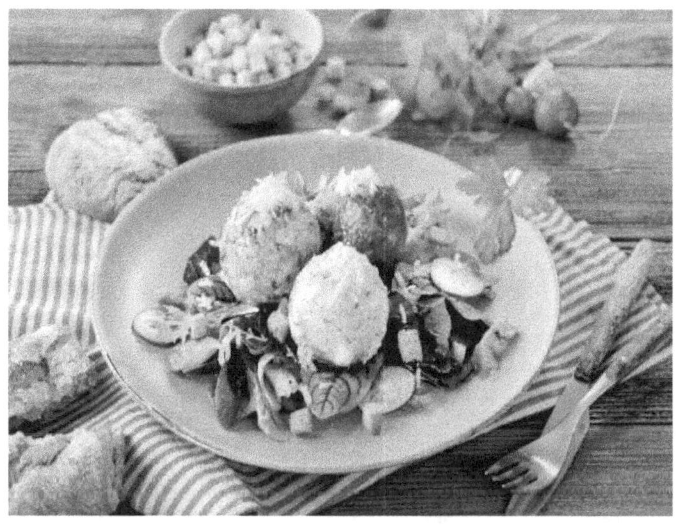

Flavorful and Nutrient-Packed Recipes for Expecting Moms

Kathleen Carrell

Table of Contents

Introduction

Once upon a time, in the quiet town of Greenfield, a radiant young woman named Cynthia found herself on the enchanting journey of motherhood. Excitement filled the air as Cynthia and her partner eagerly anticipated the arrival of their bundle of joy. However, as a first-time mom, Cynthia felt a mix of joy and trepidation about the impending changes to her life, especially when it came to nourishing herself and her growing baby. Determined to embark on a healthy and fulfilling pregnancy, Cynthia stumbled upon a gem that would become her guiding light : the "Pregnancy Diet Cookbook for Beginners." This cookbook, filled with a treasure trove of nutritious recipes tailored for expectant mothers, became Cynthia's trusted companion on her odyssey through pregnancy. The first trimester brought about waves of morning sickness, leaving Cynthia searching for gentle yet nourishing meals. Turning to the cookbook, she discovered a plethora of delightful options that eased her queasiness and provided the vital nutrients her body and baby needed. As her journey progressed into the second trimester, Cynthia's appetite soared. The cookbook's creative recipes, designed with the health of both mom and baby in mind, offered a perfect balance of proteins, whole grains, and colorful vegetables. From delectable smoothies to hearty salads, Cynthia relished every bite, knowing she was fostering a strong foundation for her baby's well-being. In the final trimester, Cynthia faced the challenges of fatigue and the occasional bout of sleeplessness. With the cookbook's guidance, she crafted meals that not only fueled her energy but also promoted relaxation. Warm, comforting dishes became a nightly ritual, helping Cynthia prepare both physically and mentally for the upcoming arrival. As Cynthia flipped through the pages of the cookbook, she found not just recipes but a supportive friend, guiding her through the perplexity and burst of pregnancy cravings and nutritional needs. She marveled at how this culinary companion made her pregnancy journey more enjoyable and empowered her to make informed, health-conscious choices. When the long-awaited day arrived, Cynthia welcomed her beautiful baby into the world, filled with gratitude for the wonderful pregnancy experience she had cultivated. The "Pregnancy Diet Cookbook for Beginners" had not only provided nourishment but had also become a source of joy, inspiration, and a connection to the incredible journey of motherhood. Cynthia's story spread through Greenfield, inspiring other moms-to-be to embark on their own healthy pregnancy journeys with the guidance of a cookbook that had turned an ordinary pregnancy into an extraordinary and flavorful adventure.

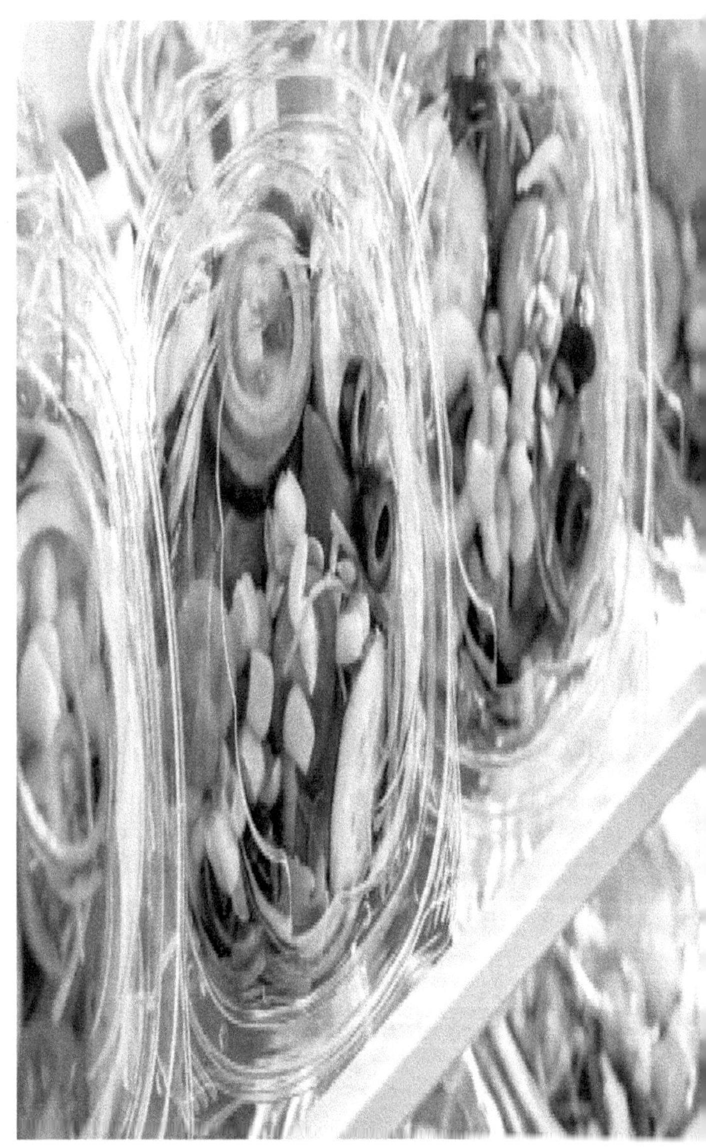

20 Balanced Breakfast for Mom and Baby's Growth

1.Oatmeal with Berries

Top a bowl of oatmeal with fresh berries for added antioxidants.

2. Greek Yogurt Parfait:

Layer Greek yogurt with granola and sliced fruits for a nutritious parfait.

3. Whole Grain Toast with Avocado:

Spread mashed avocado on whole-grain toast for a dose of healthy fats.

4. Egg and Veggie Scramble:

Scramble eggs with diced vegetables like spinach, tomatoes, and bell peppers.

5. Smoothie Bowl:

Blend your favorite fruits with yogurt, and top with nuts and seeds.

6. Chia Seed Pudding:

Mix chia seeds with milk and let it sit overnight; top with fruits in the morning.

7. Whole Wheat Pancakes:

Make pancakes using whole wheat flour and serve with a side of fruit.

8. Cottage Cheese with Pineapple:

Combine cottage cheese with fresh pineapple chunks for a protein-packed option.

9. Quinoa Breakfast Bowl:

Cook quinoa and top with nuts, dried fruits, and a drizzle of honey.

10. Banana and Peanut Butter Smoothie:

Blend bananas with peanut butter and milk for a quick and tasty smoothie.

11. Sweet Potato Hash:

Sauté sweet potatoes with onions and spinach for a hearty breakfast hash.

12. Homemade Granola Bars:

Bake your own granola bars with oats, nuts, and dried fruits.

13. Fruit Salad with Mint:

Mix a variety of seasonal fruits and add a touch of fresh mint.

14. Vegetable Frittata:

Bake eggs with a medley of vegetables for a nutrient-rich frittata.

15. Blueberry Muffins with Almond Flour:

Bake muffins using almond flour and fresh blueberries.

16. Peanut Butter Banana Toast:

Spread peanut butter on whole-grain toast and add banana slices.

17. Savory Overnight Oats:

Mix oats with yogurt, diced tomatoes, and herbs for a savory twist.

18. Cranberry Walnut Scones:

Bake scones with whole wheat flour, cranberries, and walnuts.

19. Mango and Coconut Chia Pudding:

Combine chia seeds, coconut milk, and diced mango for a tropical pudding.

20. Spinach and Feta Omelet:

Make an omelet with spinach and feta cheese for a protein boost.

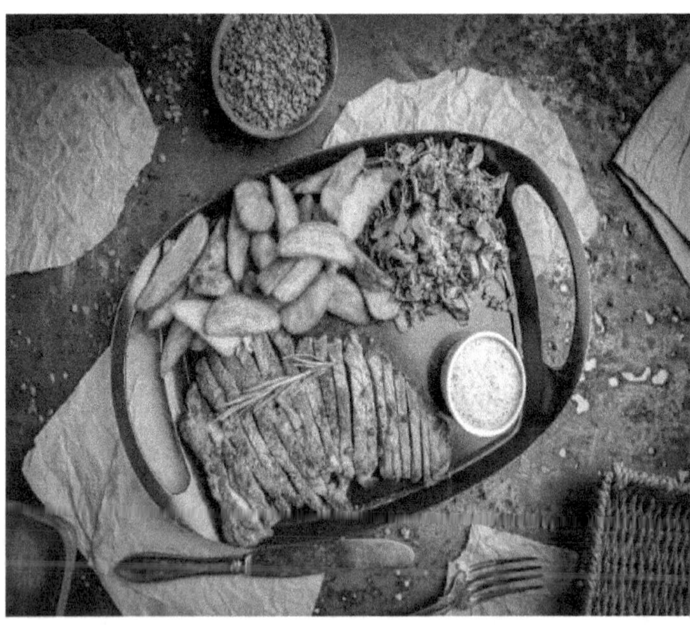

20 Balanced Lunch for Mom and Baby's Growth

1.Quinoa Salad with Chickpeas:

A protein-packed salad with quinoa, chickpeas, cherry tomatoes, cucumber, and a lemon vinaigrette.

2. Grilled Chicken Wraps:

Whole-grain wraps filled with grilled chicken, mixed greens, and a light yogurt-based dressing.

3. Salmon and Sweet Potato Bowl:

Baked salmon with roasted sweet potatoes, steamed broccoli, and a drizzle of olive oil.

4. Vegetarian Stir-Fry:

Colorful stir-fried vegetables with tofu or tempeh are served over brown rice.

5. Mediterranean Quinoa Bowl:

Quinoa topped with cherry tomatoes, feta cheese, olives, and a balsamic vinaigrette.

6. Turkey and Avocado Wrap:

Sliced turkey breast, avocado, lettuce, and tomato are wrapped in a whole-grain tortilla.

7. Greek Salad with Grilled Shrimp:

A refreshing Greek salad paired with grilled shrimp and a lemon-oregano dressing.

8. Vegetable and Lentil Soup:

A hearty soup made with lentils, various vegetables, and a tomato-based broth.

9. Whole Grain Pasta Primavera:

Whole-grain pasta tossed with a medley of sautéed vegetables and a light olive oil sauce.

10. Chicken and Quinoa Stuffed Bell Peppers:

Bell peppers stuffed with a mixture of quinoa, ground chicken, black beans, and spices.

11. Sweet Potato and Carrot Puree:

A smooth puree of roasted sweet potatoes and carrots for a vitamin A boost.

12. Avocado and Banana Mash:

Mashed avocado and banana provide healthy fats and natural sweetness.

13. Peas and Brown Rice Medley:

Soft-cooked peas are mixed with brown rice for a fiber-rich combination.

14. Broccoli and Cheddar Quinoa:

Quinoa is mixed with finely chopped broccoli and a sprinkle of mild cheddar cheese.

15. Apple and Cinnamon Oatmeal:

Steel-cut oats cooked with diced apples and a pinch of cinnamon.

16. Spinach and Lentil Puree:

Pureed spinach and lentils for a dose of iron and essential nutrients.

17. Pumpkin and Greek Yogurt Blend:

Blended pumpkin puree with Greek yogurt for a creamy and nutritious treat.

18. Chicken and Sweet Potato Mash:

Mashed sweet potatoes are combined with finely shredded cooked chicken.

19. Blueberry and Quinoa Porridge:

Quinoa porridge with blueberries is rich in antioxidants and fiber.

20. Butternut Squash and Pear Puree:

Smooth puree of roasted butternut squash and ripe pears for a sweet touch.

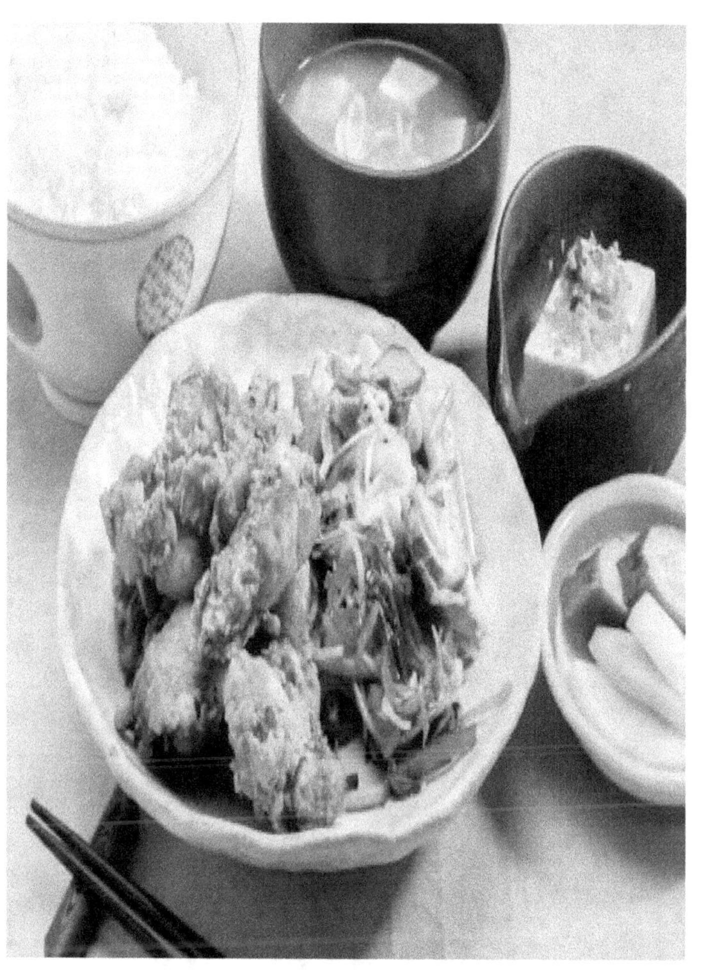

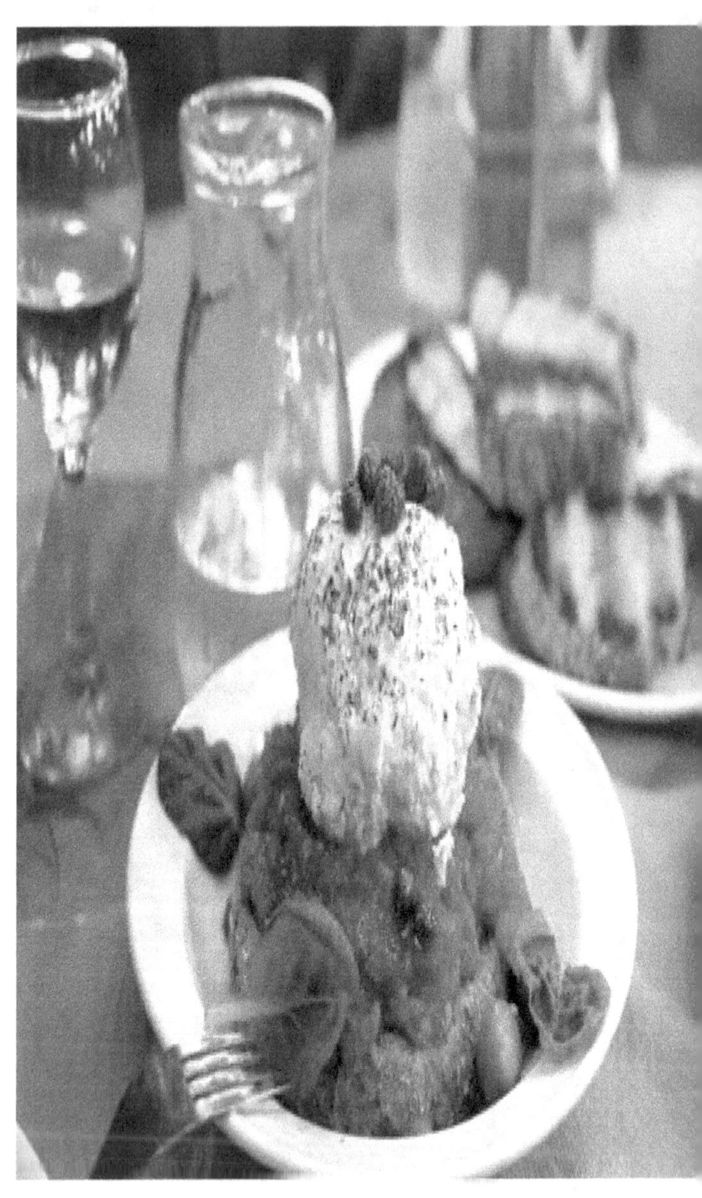

20 Balanced Dinner for Mom and Baby's Growth

1.Grilled Salmon with Quinoa:

Description: Grilled salmon provides omega-3 fatty acids crucial for a baby's brain development, paired with quinoa for a protein and fiber boost.

2. Sweet Potato and Chickpea Stew:

Description: A hearty stew combining sweet potatoes and chickpeas offers a wholesome mix of vitamins and minerals important for both mom and baby.

3. Chicken and Vegetable Stir-Fry:

Description: A colorful stir-fry with lean chicken and a variety of vegetables provides essential nutrients for both mom's and baby's growth.

4. Spinach and Feta Stuffed Chicken Breast:

Description: This dish combines lean protein from chicken with the iron and calcium-rich goodness of spinach and feta for a nutritious dinner.

5. Turkey and Quinoa Meatballs with Tomato Sauce:

Description: Turkey and quinoa meatballs are a tasty source of protein, paired with a tomato sauce rich in lycopene and vitamins.

6. Vegetarian Lentil Curry:

Description: A flavorful lentil curry provides plant-based protein, iron, and fiber, supporting the nutritional needs of both mom and baby.

7. Salmon and Asparagus Foil Packets:

Description: Easy to prepare, foil packets with salmon and asparagus offer a delicious blend of omega-3s, protein, and essential vitamins.

8. Baked Chicken with Sweet Potatoes and Broccoli:

Description: Baked chicken with sweet potatoes and broccoli provides a well-rounded mix of lean protein, complex carbs, and essential nutrients.

9. Quinoa and Black Bean Bowl:

Description: A quinoa and black bean bowl delivers a protein-packed, plant-based meal loaded with fiber, vitamins, and minerals.

10. Mushroom and spinach Whole Wheat Pasta:

Description: Whole wheat pasta with a mushroom and spinach sauce offers a nutritious combination of fiber, iron, and vitamins.

11. Tofu and Vegetable Skewers:

Description: Skewers with tofu and colorful veggies provide a plant-based protein source along with various vitamins and minerals.

12. Beef and Vegetable Stir-Fry with Brown Rice:

Description: A beef and vegetable stir-fry served with brown rice ensures a balanced mix of protein, fiber, and essential nutrients.

13. Cauliflower and Chickpea Curry:

Description: A curry with cauliflower and chickpeas offers a delightful blend of flavors and plant-based proteins for a nutritious dinner.

14. Avocado salad

Description: A refreshing salad with shrimp and avocado provides healthy fats, protein, and essential nutrients for both mom and baby.

15. Eggplant and Zucchini Lasagna:

Description: A twist on traditional lasagna, this dish with eggplant and zucchini layers is rich in antioxidants and vitamins.

16. Turkey and Vegetable Quiche:

Description: A turkey and vegetable quiche combines protein, veggies, and calcium, making it a well-rounded dinner for mom and baby.

17. Lentil and Vegetable Soup:

Description: A hearty lentil and vegetable soup is a great source of plant-based protein, fiber, and essential vitamins.

18. Grilled Chicken and Quinoa Salad:

Description: Grilled chicken paired with quinoa in a salad provides a light and nutritious dinner with a mix of proteins and whole grains.

19. Pumpkin and Lentil Stew:

Description: A pumpkin and lentil stew offers a flavorful combination of plant-based protein, fiber, and essential nutrients.

20. Cottage Cheese and Fruit Parfait:

Description: A parfait with cottage cheese and mixed fruits is a light and refreshing option, providing protein, vitamins, and minerals.

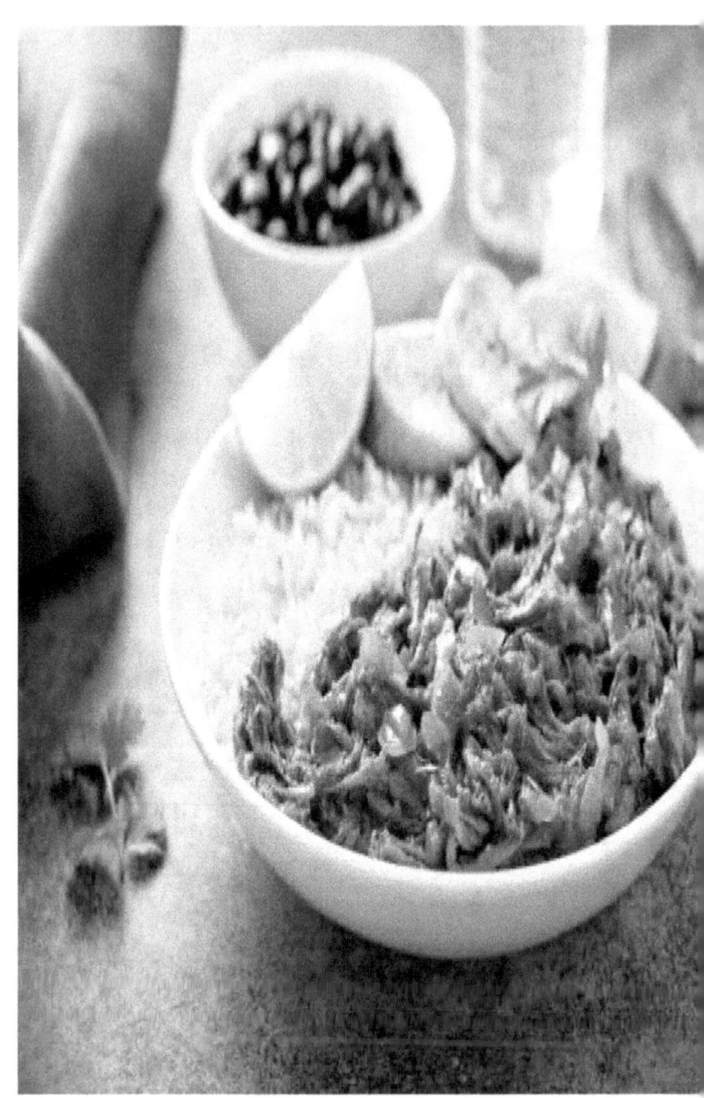

10 Healthy Snacks for a Mom to be wellness

1.Trail Mix Bliss:

Combine a mix of raw nuts, seeds, and dried fruits for a crunchy and energy-boosting snack that provides essential nutrients.

2. Greek Yogurt Parfait:

Layer Greek yogurt with fresh berries and a drizzle of honey for a protein-rich and delicious treat that promotes a healthy pregnancy.

3. Hummus and Veggie Sticks:

Dive into a bowl of hummus paired with colorful vegetable sticks for a fiber-packed snack that satisfies cravings and supports digestion.

4. Avocado Toast Delight:

Spread mashed avocado on whole-grain toast and sprinkle with a pinch of sea salt for a tasty snack loaded with healthy fats.

5. Chia Pudding Power:

Create a chia seed pudding with almond milk and top it with sliced fruits for a nutrient-dense snack that's rich in omega-3 fatty acids.

6. Protein-Packed Cottage Cheese:

Enjoy a bowl of cottage cheese with a sprinkle of nuts or seeds for a high-protein snack that aids in muscle development.

7. Fruit Smoothie Boost:

Blend together your favorite fruits with yogurt and a handful of spinach for a refreshing and vitamin-packed smoothie.

8. Nut Butter Banana Bites:

Spread almond or peanut butter on banana slices for a tasty and satisfying snack that combines healthy fats and potassium.

9. Whole Grain Crackers with Cheese:

Pair whole grain crackers with a serving of cheese for a calcium-rich snack that supports bone health during pregnancy.

10. Roasted Chickpeas Crunch:

Roast chickpeas with a blend of spices for a crunchy snack that delivers protein and iron essential for a healthy pregnancy.

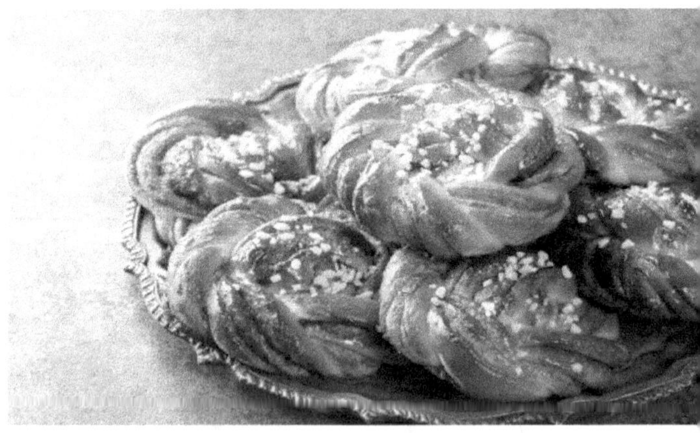

10 Healthy Smoothie and Benefits for a Mom to be wellness

1.Berry Bliss Smoothie:

Ingredients: mixed berries (strawberries, blueberries, raspberries), Greek yogurt, almond milk, chia seeds, honey.

Benefits: rich in antioxidants, fiber, and calcium for bone health.

2. Green Goddess Glow:

Ingredients: spinach, banana, avocado, pineapple, and coconut water.

Benefits: Packed with folate, potassium, and vitamins for a healthy pregnancy glow.

3. Pregnancy Power Protein Smoothie:

Ingredients: almond butter, banana, Greek yogurt, milk, and flaxseeds.

Benefits: high protein content for energy and muscle support.

4. Citrus Burst Delight:

Ingredients: oranges, mango, plain yogurt, carrots, and ginger.

Benefits: Vitamin C for immune support and digestion aid.

5. Nutty Banana Boost:

Ingredients: almond milk, banana, walnuts, dates, and cinnamon.

Benefits: Provides essential omega-3 fatty acids and iron for energy.

6. Prenatal Green Kiwi Cooler:

Ingredients: Kiwi, kale, cucumber, mint leaves, coconut water.

Benefits: rich in vitamin K, C, and hydrating properties.

7. Antioxidant Avocado Elixir:

Ingredients: avocado, blueberries, kale, lime juice, water.

Benefits: It supports healthy brain development and the immune system.

8. Mango Tango Smoothie:

Ingredients: mango, plain yogurt, almond milk, chia seeds, honey.

Benefits: Vitamin A and fiber for healthy skin and digestion.

9. Calcium-Rich Almond Fig Fantasy:

Ingredients: figs, almond milk, Greek yogurt, flaxseeds, honey.

Benefits: It boosts calcium intake for bone health.

10. Pineapple Coconut Bliss:

Ingredients: pineapple, coconut milk, banana, spinach, and ice.

Benefits: refreshing and hydrating, with a tropical twist.

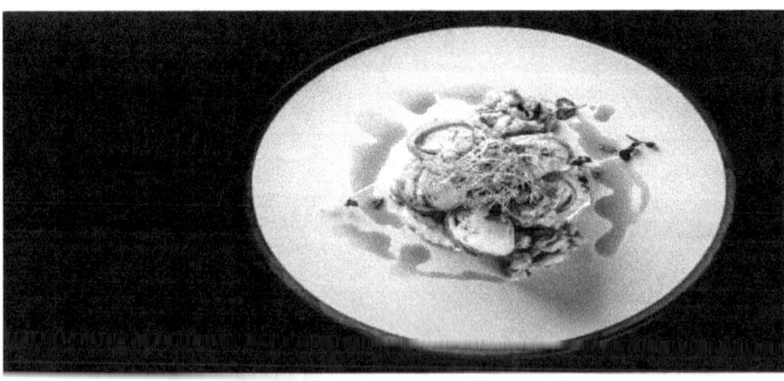

7 days Meal Plan for an expecting Moms

Day 1:

Breakfast:

- Whole-grain toast with avocado
- Poached eggs
- Fresh fruit salad

Lunch:

- Grilled chicken salad with mixed greens and vinaigrette
- Quinoa on the side
- Greek yogurt with berries

Dinner:

- Baked salmon
- Sweet potato wedges
- Steamed broccoli

Snack:

- Almonds and a piece of cheese

Day 2:

Breakfast:

- Smoothie with spinach, banana, almond milk, and chia seeds
- Whole-grain muffin

Lunch:

- Lentil soup
- Whole-grain roll
- Mixed fruit bowl

Dinner:

- Stir-fried tofu with vegetables
- Brown rice
- Sliced mango for dessert

Snack:

- Greek yogurt with a drizzle of honey

Day 3:

Breakfast:

- Overnight oats with almond milk, topped with nuts and berries
- Hard-boiled egg

Lunch:

- Turkey and avocado wrap with a whole-grain tortilla
- Carrot and cucumber sticks with hummus

Dinner:

- Quinoa-stuffed bell peppers
- Grilled shrimp skewers
- Steamed asparagus

Snack:

- Apple slices with peanut butter

<u>**Day 4:**</u>

Breakfast:

- Whole-grain pancakes with Greek yogurt and sliced strawberries
- Orange juice

Lunch:

- Caprese salad with whole-grain crackers
- Lentil and vegetable stew

Dinner:

- Baked chicken breast
- Quinoa pilaf with roasted vegetables
- Fresh pineapple chunks

Snack:

- Handful of mixed nuts

Day 5:

Breakfast:

- Oatmeal with sliced bananas and almonds
- Glass of orange juice

Lunch:

- Grilled chicken salad with mixed greens, cherry tomatoes, and balsamic vinaigrette
- Whole-grain roll

Dinner:

- Baked salmon with lemon and dill
- Quinoa pilaf
- Steamed broccoli

Snack:

- Greek yogurt with a sprinkle of chia seeds

Day 6:

Breakfast:

- Whole-grain toast with mashed avocado
- Scrambled eggs with spinach
- Fresh berries

Lunch:

- Lentil and vegetable soup
- Whole-grain crackers
- Mixed fruit salad

Dinner:

- Stir-fried tofu with broccoli and brown rice
- Sliced mango for dessert

Snack:

- A handful of almonds

Day 7:

Breakfast:

- Smoothie with kale, banana, and almond milk
- Whole-grain muffin

Lunch:

- Turkey and vegetable wrap with a whole-grain tortilla
- Carrot and cucumber sticks with hummus

Dinner:

- Grilled shrimp skewers
- Quinoa salad with cherry tomatoes and avocado
- Steamed asparagus

Snack:

- Cottage cheese with pineapple chunks

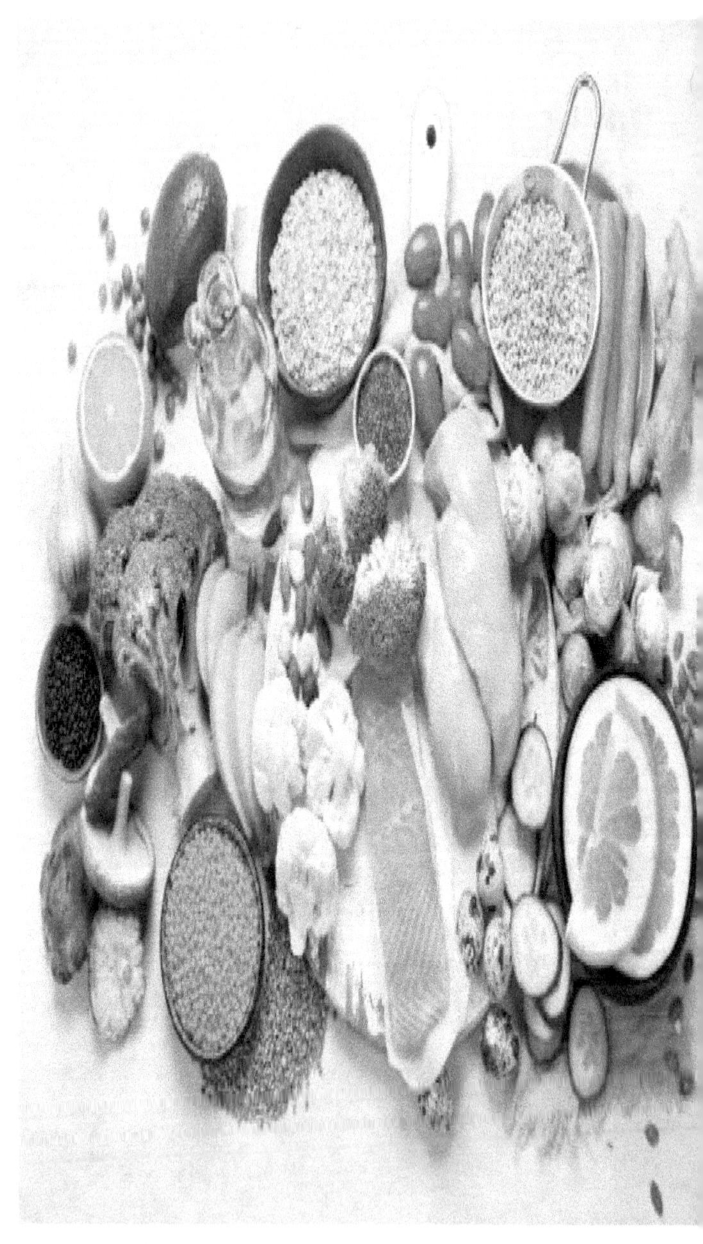

Conclusion

Firstly, I want to express my heartfelt gratitude for choosing "Nourishing Beginnings: A Pregnancy Diet Cookbook for Beginners." Your journey into parenthood is a unique and beautiful experience, and I am honored to be a part of it through this cookbook. In this guide, we've embarked on a culinary journey tailored to support you during this incredible phase of life. From nutritious recipes designed to meet the needs of both you and your growing baby to practical tips on maintaining a balanced pregnancy diet, I trust this cookbook has been a valuable companion on your path to a healthy pregnancy. As you savor the delicious recipes and incorporate the recommended nutrients into your daily meals, remember that each dish is crafted with care and consideration for both taste and well-being. Your health is of utmost importance, and I hope this cookbook has empowered you with the knowledge and inspiration needed to make informed choices throughout your pregnancy. Thank you for allowing me to be a part of your pregnancy journey. I wish you health, joy, and a smooth transition into this new chapter of your life.

Warm regards,

Your Favorite Dietitian **Kathleen Carrell!!**

www.ingramcontent.com/pod-product-compliance
Lightning Source LLC
Chambersburg PA
CBHW071128260726
48661CB00006B/2716